About Black Hair

by

R.L. Worthy

KornerStone Books
6947 Coal Creek Pkwy

Published by

KornerStone Books
6947 Coal Creek Pkwy
Suite 206
Newcastle, WA 98059
Ksbooks@execs.com

Editor: Ethel Williams Thompson

Design and Layout: KornerStone Books

Images courtesy of The Hall of Records - Kornerstone ©

Printed in the United States of America

The First Edition

ISBN: 0-9727627-5-2

If you will know yourselves, then you will be known and you will know that you are the children of the Living Father. But if you do not know yourselves, then you are in poverty and you are poverty . . .

Yeshua Ham-Mashiach

Introduction

A recent study on the health of African Americans has brought a rather appalling fact to the fore. Incredibly, millions of African American women are losing their hair. What's even more remarkable about this finding is that it's the conditioned behavior of many of these women that's causing them to experience this misfortune.

The study explains that the pursuit of "American Beauty" (i.e., to have straight hair) is actually proving detrimental to the health and condition of the hair of African American women. In truth, these clinicians are reiterating facts that have been known by many for years; i.e., that tight braids, ponytails or extensions, bonding glue, chemical relaxers, and the layering of multiple hair treatments is harmful and has led to the balding of millions of African American women. The study goes on to reveal that this self-manufactured baldness is leading to lowered self-esteem and serious depression for many of these African American women as well.

As a student of history, I am well aware that any Black infatuation with having straight hair is a late phenomenon. Therefore, I have little choice but to address this modern day predicament of my sistren. The obvious quandary being—*the harder they try, the further they fall behind* . . .

However, at the outset let me say that I won't be brow-beating African American women for sho'nuff not wanting to have "Nappy-Hair." Rather, I shall attempt to bring some perspective to the subject of Black hair. Accordingly, I shall employ four spheres of study in this book; i.e., history, anatomy, spirituality, and psychology.

In closing, it is my hope that the ensuing pages *about Black hair* will not only prove life affirming—but useful . . .

CONTENTS

CONTENTS

Reader's Guide to the Work

Though trying to create a no frills straightforward document, I have been forced to employ the use of two time and space saving reference symbols: Roman numerals and the word net in parentheses (net).

A Roman numeral at the end of a sentence indicates reference cites and more information about the subject. The cite can be found in the corresponding endnote located at the end of the text.

The term <u>net</u> in parentheses (net) at the end of a citation has been used to indicate that the reference was found on the Internet. The precise url (website address) and date of the source can be found in the bibliography.

History

Some will ask, What could world history possibly have to do with having healthy Black hair? Here is my answer: Forasmuch as 99.9% of the discussion about Black people in the West (after the 15th century) revolves around some fair to middling response to an intellectual, cultural, or physical assault by Whites—it is clear that it is impossible to undertake an honest and meaningful examination of the "Black Character" without considering those cultures whose experience was not adulterated by the ardent racism that permeates these times. To this end, I shall concentrate most of my attention upon the ancient Black peoples of the Fertile Crescent.

While I will focus upon the ancient Africans of the Nile Valley, I shall also touch upon the Black Hamitic and Shemitic peoples of Western Asia. I should think that my rationale here is manifest insomuch as no Black societies in history were more culturally intact than the civilizations that flourished in the Fertile Crescent before the emergence of the Caucasian in the region.

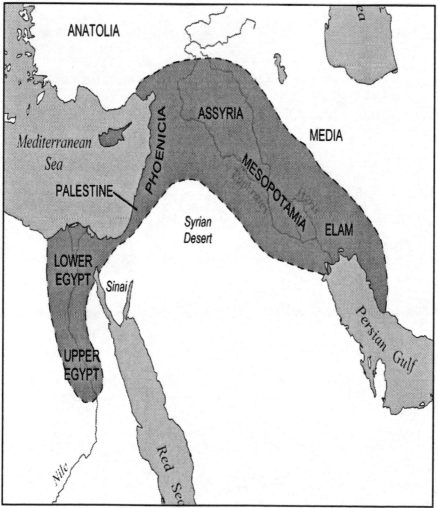

Map of the Fertile Crescent

Black Hair
in the
Fertile Crescent

Black Hair in the Fertile Crescent

As previously alluded to, the Fertile Crescent was first inhabited by Black Hamites and Shemites (Shemite back cover). Yet, in that no people (Black or White) has ever been more spiritual, accomplished, compassionate, or self-assured about their place in creation than the Egyptians—I can think of no better place to begin our discussion than with the Africans of the Nile Valley.

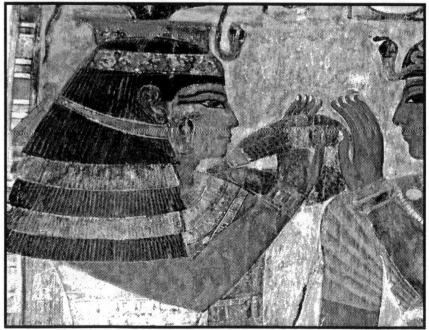

Isis & Seti c.1100 BC

To begin, the biological purpose of the hair is to provide protection from the sun, weather, and light surface blows to the head. Of course, the woolly hair of the Black Race performs these tasks quite well! In addition, hair has long been held as a facet of one's general health and sexual allure. There is incontrovertible evidence that the Black peoples of the Fertile Crescent grew and treasured their hair. Conversely, amongst these people the close cut (or shaved) head was seen as representing someone in mourning, captivity, or slavery.[1]

---

[1] Hair, Great Soviet Encyclopedia Vol. V, pp. 182 -183 & Hairdressing, The American Peoples Encyclopedia Vol. X, p. 107 & Budge, E.A., The Dwellers on the Nile p. 256 & Muller, M., Mythology of All Races Vol. XII, p. 193 & Higgins, G., Anacalypsis Vol. II, pp. 78 - 79 & Ancient Mesopotamia p. 25 & Herm, G., The Phoenicians p. 199 & & Owen, F., The Germanic People p. 117
For certain priestly sects, a close cut had religious significance. However, in most instances, to grasp or cut someone's hair was symbolic of their total loss and submission. Owen explains that even amongst the ancient Germanic peoples of Europe, long hair was a symbol of noble birth. Moreover, people with short hair were not only considered of lower class—but as long as their hair was short they could not rise in status.

Black Hair in the Fertile Crescent

In actual point of fact, it was customary for the ancient Egyptians to wear their natural locking hair rather long by today's standards. The ancient Persians were even to comment about the long natural hairstyles of many of the people of the Nile Valley. Indeed, one of the clearest expressions of the ancient Egyptians' respect for their Black identity was the regard they had for the natural character of their hair (but a bit more about that later).

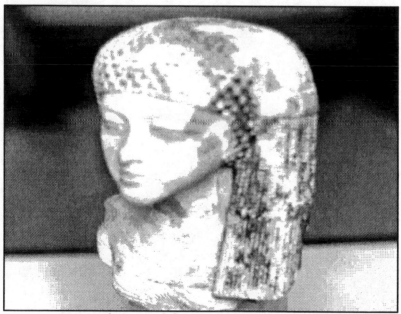

Egyptian Noble Women c.1400 BC

Wigs

<u>Wigs</u>

I am aware that some Caucasian writers have told you that most Egyptians kept their heads shaved and routinely wore wigs throughout their daily lives—<u>that's false</u>! Having personally viewed the artifacts of many Egyptian tombs, it is true that from time to time one can find wigs made of sheep's wool. However, this is probably because the individual buried in that particular tomb had aged and was not particularly happy with his (or her) own head of hair—or should I say the lack of it. But the fact that some Egyptians naturally went bald does not mean that we should conclude that everyone in Egypt was unable, or did not desire, to grow their own hair.

As for those priestly orders in ancient Egypt who kept their heads shaved, this practice was not a rejection of their hair or suggest a people's desire to be bald. Rather, it is emblematic of one of the sacred obligations of a particular spiritual order. In fact, it is not difficult to conversely find orders of Egyptian priests who were to grow their hair quite long.

Even more here, if the truth is to be told, the people of the Nile are known to have tried to create hair-growing salves (out of certain animal fats) for people who were going bald. This was most probably attempted because, then as now, a healthy head of hair was associated with youth, vigor and virility. Yet, the real point here is that the Blacks of the Nile would not have spent their time and energy trying to create a medicine to grow the hair of the elderly, and/or balding, if they had some cultural aversion to possessing it!

Furthermore, we know that, then as now, a favorite pastime of Egyptian women was to gather together and spend long sessions styling their hair.[1] However, no credible Egyptologist believes these women were spending this time styling wigs for daily wearing. Obviously, any suggestion that this female gymnast is wearing a wig is simply nonsense. Thus, nothing could be clearer; the substitution of a wig for real hair was not a desirable circumstance for the lovely Black women of ancient Egypt.

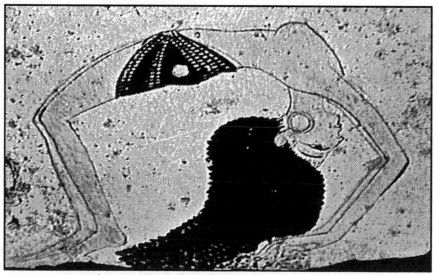

Ancient Egyptian Gymnast c.1200 BC

---

[1] I Corinthians 11:15
While we're on the subject, some of you may even recall the ancient scripture that explains that long hair is to a woman's glory. FYI: the original language of this instruction was Black—connect the dots if you dare.

This all said, the simplest way to disprove the life long wig-wearer notion is the fact that many Egyptian renderings depict old men with relatively long locked hair on the sides and back of their heads—yet, with none on top. Of course, these portraits are illustrations of Egyptians who had classic male baldness. Or, are we now to believe that the Egyptians made wigs that only covered the back and sides of a man's head?[2]

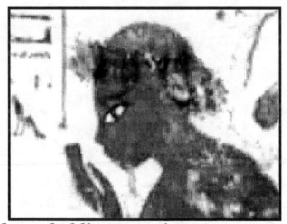

Locks on balding Egyptian Man c.1400 BC

---

[2] Mertz, B., <u>Red Land, Black Land</u> p. 79 & Bullock, M., <u>Daily Life in Ancient Egypt</u> & Boorstin, D., <u>The Discoverers</u> p. 147 & Budge, E.A., <u>The Dwellers on the Nile</u> p. 69 & Ghalioungui, P., <u>Magic and Medical Science in ancient Egypt</u> p. 153 & Lucas, A., <u>Ancient Egyptian Materials & Industry</u> p. 383

In passing, the fat of the lion and of black snakes were two (of the many) elements that were used in Egyptian cures.

Locks

Having come to understand that the ancient Blacks of the Nile were to embrace, not reject, their God-given physiology—we actually find the significance of their hair being manifold. You see, not being at odds with themselves, Blacks of the Old World would not merely grow their hair for vanity's sake—it was also considered an extension of their spiritual and material being! As a matter of fact, it is no stretch to analogize that just as the rings of a tree trunk mark its age—the ancients saw their hair as a testament (or record) of their life experience. In other words, the chapters of a life being expressed in the ringlets of hair emitted from the scalp and ultimately transformed into locks (or columns) of wool.[1]

---

[1] Dampier-Whetham, W., <u>A History Of Science: And its relations with Philosophy & Religion</u> p. xxvii
It's noteworthy here that hair is one of the anatomical substances scientists test to determine what chemicals have been put into the <u>material</u> body. You might say its used to reveal past deeds—hmmm', kinda like a record.

Locks

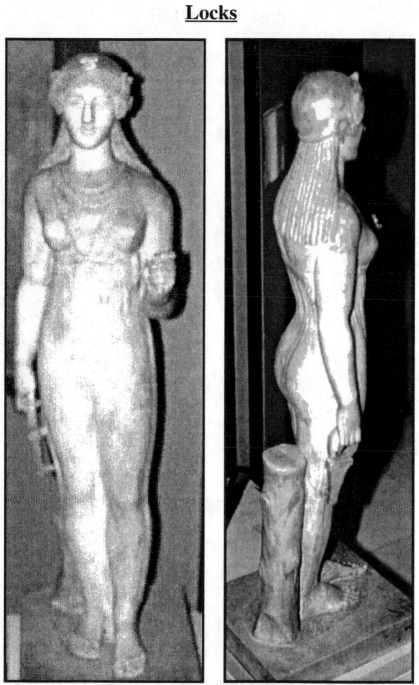

This life size lock wearing Goddess represents the Mother of the Black peoples of the Nile c.300 BC

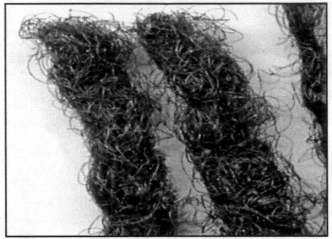

Here's what the terrifying natural locks of a Black person actually look like. <u>Thickness is a personal choice</u>; for instance, many of the Blacks of the ancient Mediterranean wore them (uniformly) about the circumference of a finger. In Egypt, however, they were often worn thinner (about the circumference of a pencil).

Allow me to take a moment to share a few examples of the important, and even spiritual properties, that were attributed to the hair by Blacks throughout the ancient Fertile Crescent and Mediterranean:

- Egyptian legend tells us that Ra created women from one lock of his hair.

- Osiris vowed that no lock should be cut from his head before returning home to Egypt from

Locks

Ethiopia.

- We learn that upon hearing about the death of her husband Osiris, Isis cut one of her locks. This is probably why the Egyptian people are known to have cut their locks in times of misfortune or great loss. A lock of Queen Tiye's hair is said to have been placed in the tomb of Tutankhamen.

- Ancient Egyptian pyramid texts speak of the great God who grips the locks on the top of the head.

- Egyptian depictions of a king or queen cutting an adversary's hair symbolized the enemy's total subjugation.

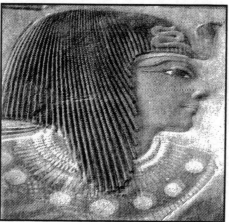

Side locks of Egyptian Nobleman c.1100 BC

- Incidentally, in Egypt the frontal side locks were often worn a bit longer. Gaskell contends that the peoples of the Old (or <u>First</u>) World considered the side locks to represent, or possibly facilitate, the attainment of spiritual intuition.

- The spiritual significance of hair was not wasted on Egypt's neighbors. For instance, the celebrated Babylonian tale of <u>The Epic of Gilamesh</u> clearly associates the length of the hero Enkidu's hair with his great physical strength.

- In Hebraic scripture we find: *"All the days of the vow of his separation there shall no razor come upon his head: until the days be fulfilled, in which he separateth himself unto the Lord, he shall be holy, and shall let the locks of the hair of his head grow."* The scriptures also state: *"For, lo, thou shalt conceive and bear a son; and no razor shall come upon his head: for the child shall be a Nazarite unto God from the womb."*

- The Septuagint Bible tells us how Sampson's strength, and demise, was directly related to to the length of his hair. After being duped by Delilah (whose name fittingly means "She who makes Weak") Samson's strength was sapped when she cut his seven locks.

- The scriptures also explain that the wise King

Locks

Solomon wore locks. And scholars of Judaic culture tell us that the hair of the unfaithful woman was commonly cut off.

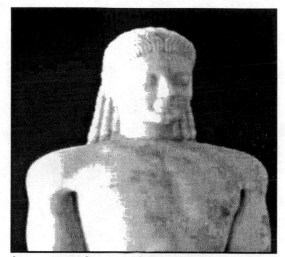

This is an ancient Minoan Man c.2000 BC

- Coming down to the era of the ancient Greeks, in a rather familiar account, the kingdom of Nisus was conquered after the king lost his hair. Like Samson, King Nisus and his throne were considered to be invincible as long as he had a long lock of hair. Tricking Princess Scylla into betraying her father to prove her love for him, King Minos had Scylla cut her father's purple lock. Once lockless, Nisus was defenseless against the Minoans. Shortly thereafter, his kingdom was destroyed.

- Some chronicles cite instances of women

dedicating a lock of hair to their lovers as a demonstration of their devotion to them.

- Christian scripture explains that the beloved Child of the Promise" has hair *"like wool."*

- The ancient Hyperboreans cut their locks at times of mourning.

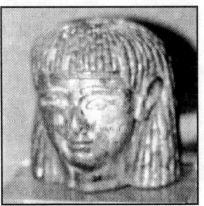

This is a Phoenician Man in locks. They were cousins of the ancient Hebrews who also wore locks.

- Lastly, as touched upon, the hair was not only seen as a receptor for spiritual and physical power, it has even been considered to be a sacred record of the life! Interestingly, a passage in <u>Ezekiel</u> explains:
"For what is a lock of the head but the thoughts of the mind gathered together, so as not to be scattered and dispersed, but to remain bound by discipline. A hand is therefore put forth from above, and the prophet is lifted up by the lock of his head."[i]

To begin, the biological purpose of the hair is to provide protection from the sun, weather, and light surface blows to the head. Of course, the woolly hair of the Black Race performs these tasks quite well! In addition, hair has long been held as a facet of one's general health and sexual allure. There is incontrovertible evidence that the Black peoples of the Fertile Crescent grew and treasured their hair. Conversely, amongst these people the close cut (or shaved) head was seen as representing someone in mourning, captivity, or slavery.[1]

---

[1] Hair, Great Soviet Encyclopedia Vol. V, pp. 182 -183 & Hairdressing, The American Peoples Encyclopedia Vol. X, p. 107 & Budge, E.A., The Dwellers on the Nile p. 256 & Muller, M., Mythology of All Races Vol. XII, p. 193 & Higgins, G., Anacalypsis Vol. II, pp. 78 - 79 & Ancient Mesopotamia p. 25 & Herm, G., The Phoenicians p. 199 & & Owen, F., The Germanic People p. 117
For certain priestly sects, a close cut had religious significance. However, in most instances, to grasp or cut someone's hair was symbolic of their total loss and submission. Owen explains that even amongst the ancient Germanic peoples of Europe, long hair was a symbol of noble birth. Moreover, people with short hair were not only considered of lower class—but as long as their hair was short they could not rise in status.

Black Hair in the Fertile Crescent

As previously alluded to, the Fertile Crescent was first inhabited by Black Hamites and Shemites (Shemite back cover). Yet, in that no people (Black or White) has ever been more spiritual, accomplished, compassionate, or self-assured about their place in creation than the Egyptians—I can think of no better place to begin our discussion than with the Africans of the Nile Valley.

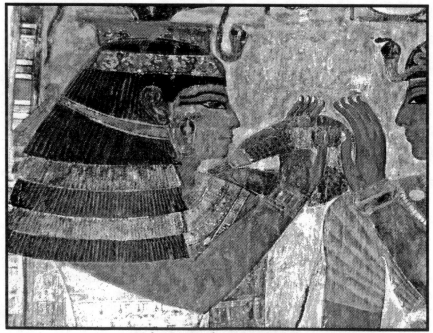

Isis & Seti c.1100 BC

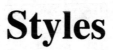

Styles

To briefly address the hairstyles of the Egyptians, once more—<u>it was as natural for ancient black men to wear their hair in locks as it is to find Caucasians wearing it in crew-cuts today</u>. Black noblemen commonly wore their locks about shoulder length with the side locks slightly longer. The more physically active men of Egypt (e.g., soldiers, farmers, and craftsmen) generally wore their locks a bit shorter in length.[1] In passing, as for facial hair, most Egyptian males went through life clean-shaven.[2]

---

[1] Oates, J., <u>Babylon</u> p. 33 & Gray, J., <u>Near Eastern Mythology</u> p. 61 & Eban, A., <u>Heritage: Civilization and the Jews</u> p. 14 & Macaulay, R., <u>Pleasure of Ruins</u> & Wheeler, M., <u>Flames Over Persepolis</u> & Glubot, S., <u>Discovering the Royal Tombs at Ur</u> p. 65
While it is not impossible to find portrayals of ancient Blacks in Asia wearing locks, many wore their hair in a style similar to the modern Afro. That said, these Babylonians often wore their beards in a locked fashion (see back cover).
[2] Mertz, B., <u>Red Land, Black Land</u> p. 79 & (Video), <u>Ancient Lives</u> WTTW 1988 & Bullock, M., <u>Daily Life in Ancient Egypt</u> & Mialon, E., <u>The Great Pharaoh Ramses and His Time</u> Chp. 54 - 55

Styles

In that the disposition of these African women was such that their natural essence was hardly something merely embraced for a few weeks out of a year, or for a couple of years during a decade—<u>they grew and kept their locks long throughout their lives</u>; often wearing them freely down their backs! The fact that they grew their locks long also made it possible for Egyptian women to create many different hair styles; hence, the finding that they loved having their locks treated and styled. Indeed, Tertullian would state the following about the North African women's hair of his day: *"You will not let it have a moment's rest: one day it is tied back, another day it falls loose; now it is lifted high, now it is pressed flat . . ."*[3]

The profession of barber was widely practiced in Egypt. Many barbers made house calls to cut hair or shave a client. Even though razors were commonly made of bronze, they were also made of gold, silex and copper. FYI: the pic (or rake) combs found in some tombs were probably used to tend mustaches, facial, or body hair rather than locks.

[3] Budge, E.A., <u>Egypt</u> p. 33 & Mertz, B., <u>Red Land, Black Land</u> pp. 76 - 79 & Butzer, C. (Ed.), <u>Ancient Egypt:</u>

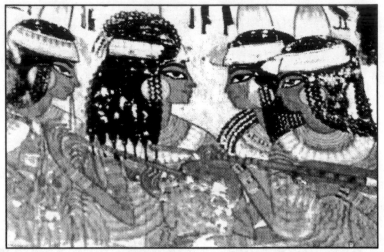

Egyptian Women during a celebration c.1200 BC

As a matter of fact, one way to distinguish the different Egyptian goddesses and queens is by the length and individual styling of their locks. Mertz writes:

> *"Ladies usually wore their black hair long . . . A popular and becoming style was to let the long hair hang loose, thick and*

Discovering Its Splendors p. 104 & Budge, E.A., The Dwellers on the Nile p. 69 & Budge, E.A., A History of Egypt Vol. I, p. 51 & Freemantle, A., A Treasury of Early Christianity p. 63 & Mertz, B., Red Land, Black Land pp. 76 - 79 & Wheelwright, E., Medicinal Plants and their History
As opposed to the poisonous chemicals used by many Blacks today—olive oil was one of the most commonly used conditioners for the locks of ancient Black people.

waving, from under a fillet or wreath of flowers; but women were not always content with such simplicity. Sometimes they braided [see footnote] their hair into many tiny plaits, or separated it into ringlets bound with gold . . ."[4]

A final point: after decades of research I have found little to suggest that Egyptian women were applying dyes to their hair to change its natural color. It seems that the vast majority of Egyptian women were quite happy with the natural hues of their locks. In truth, after years of study I've found no evidence of red or blonde

---

[4] Mertz, B., <u>Red Land, Black Land</u> p. 76
Although Mertz makes a yeoman's effort here, do not be confused by the phrase *"braided their hair"* as (being White) she is understandably not familiar with the true character of Black hair. Ancient Egyptian women did not need to braid their hair in the sense that people think of braiding today. Frankly, the general confluence in braiding is relatively vertical, while with a lock its more horizontal. Thus, <u>their hair locking naturally—these women were in fact styling their locks into many "braided" styles</u>! Egyptian men seldom chose to weave their locks into braids or put beads on them.

dyes being applied to locks! We needn't be shocked by this finding for two reasons: first, the Egyptian physiology was Black; and second, despite the fact that many of you are not aware of it, light hair was not highly regarded in many parts of the Old World. For example, as late as the life of Christ we find the Romans associating blonde hair and/or wigs with prostitution.[5]

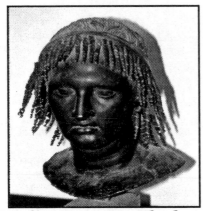 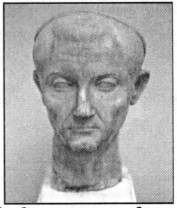

Mediterranean Black with locks worn under a headband and Caucasian of the same ancient region

---

[5] Wigs, <u>Encyclopedia Britannica</u> Vol. XXVIII, p. 624 & Simons, G., <u>Barbarian Europe</u> p. 18 & Owen, F., <u>The Germanic People</u> p. 150 & Scullard, H., <u>Roman Britain</u> p. 16 & Robinson, C., <u>Conversion of Europe</u> pp. 98 - 99
The celebrated Romans Ovid and Juvenal explain that blonde hair was associated with prostitution in Rome. This was probably because many of the first Nordic Caucasians to come to Rome would have been brought there as slaves.

Why Black Hair Locks

As for the anatomical reason why Black hair locks, we must look to the miraculous substance of melanin. Interestingly, just as the degree of activated melanin imparts different properties to the skin of the different races—it also affects the character of the hair. This is why anthropologists have long held hair to be one of the determiners of race: the amount and type of melanin in the hair determining its color and physical character.

Biologically speaking, activated melanin is the anatomical substance that produces skin color in human beings. Basically, the more activated melanin a person has, the richer the color—the less, the paler. Wills makes the following disclosure about melanin in human beings:

> *"The master enzyme in all this is tyrosinase. If the gene for this enzyme is*

defective, the result is a person with albinism, someone who makes no melanin at all. But the most remarkable discovery made by molecular biologists has been that most of us, regardless of skin color, have quite enough tyrosinase in our melanocytes to make us very black. In those of us with light skin, something is preventing the enzyme from functioning at full capacity . . ."[1]

It is obvious that Blacks have much higher concentrations of activated melanin in the epidermal layer of their skin.[2] Yet, insomuch as black skin has been so maligned in these times, allow me to take a moment to share some rather

---

[1] Wills, C., The Skin We're In Discover Nov. 15, No. 11 Nov. 1994 pp. 79 – 80 & Coon, C., Racial Adaptations pp. 48 – 49
See chapter endnote for more about activated melanin.
[2] Biological Coloration, The Encyclopedia Britannica Vol. XVI, p. 588 & Wills, C., The Skin We're In Discover Nov. 15, No. 11 Nov. 1994 p. 79

interesting facts about melanin in human beings:

- First, it is the substance of melanin that produces skin color in all healthy human life. People with the least amount of activated melanin lie in the paler spectrums. Those having the most make up the people with brown and black skin.

- Second, activated melanin is not now, nor ever has been, a recessive trait in human beings.

- Third, activated melanin absorbs the ultra-violet rays of the sun. This means that skin cells with activated melanin are able to safely absorb more heat from sunlight than those without. Moreover, activated melanin is believed to serve as a block from the harmful rays of the sun. This provides the darker races with greater protection from skin damage and melanomas (cancer) from sunlight.

- The organic chemist Carol Barnes contends that during the day melanin functions as a seratonin, while acting as an alkaloid at night. Seratonin is a derivative of the important amino acid tryptophan. Alkaloids are naturally occurring organic substances that stimulate the nervous system.

- It should be noted that kinesiology Professor Malachi Andrews believes the neuromelanin in the brain stem and cerebellum of Blacks facilitates complex and rhythmic motor functions. Also, in <u>Racial Adaptations</u> we find: *"Pigmentation varies racially in two parts of the eye. One is the outer surface of the retina . . . Rays of visual light that pass through it enter two glands in the brain that speed up or slow down the reaction of our nervous systems to stimuli. The amount of light that reaches these glands depends partly on retinal color; as a result there are racial differences in certain aspects of behavior. Pink and yellow retinas reflect light that darker ones absorb; they slow reactions down, while darker retinas speed them up."*

- The distinguished anthropologist Charleton Coon would say of sunlight and human biology:
"Tanning prepares the bare parts of the skin for the growth-stimulating effects of the ultraviolet rays that pass through the cuticle, epidermis, and corium into the underlying fatty tissue. There they encounter a cholesterol, pre-vitamin D_3 which, in turn, is

transformed into proper functional vitamin D₃ by the person's own body heat. This vitamin D₃ then meanders through the blood stream to the liver and then the kidneys. In the liver and kidneys the vitamin is converted twice by the action of hydroxide ions (OH-) into a substance that helps convert ingested minerals—calcium, phosphorus, and trace metals—into parts of the living tissue. That is how we get our bones and brains and the iron in our blood's red cells. We also gain a wide tolerance to different strengths of ultraviolet rays because of this long, multiple, and mutually compensatory sequence of metabolic and digestive processes."

The salient point here is that eumelanin (found in black and brown skin) is the greatest facilitator of the absorption of sunlight in humans.

- Permit me to say a word about the hormone melatonin. Working in conjunction with melanin, melatonin is considered to play an important role in the operations of the human biological clock. While some declare the name to be derived from the ancient terms *melas* and *tosos* meaning "black-workings," others explain that it was derivative of the Greek name *Melos-Anos*, which was the name of the

Why Black Hair Locks

Black Goddess Aphorite who was the mother of Delphos. In any event, the pineal gland is responsible for the production of this hormone. Incidentally, of the two sexes, women possess the largest pineal glands.

- Lastly here, it is clear that the ancient peoples of the Nile Valley were to cherish the color in their skin. One clear illustration of this rests in the finding that to refer to someone as a "Nubian" was, in effect, to call them a member of the gold race. [ii]

Now, as for hair and melanin, biologists explain that hair shafts are not solid structures but more like tunnels. In short, the hair is principally made up of dead cells that contain keratin (a strong fibrous protein). The part of the hair that is above the skin is called the shaft; the part below it is called the root. At the base of each hair in the dermis (skin) is its bulb. The follicle, which fulfils two important functions, encases the root and bulb. First, it contains the melanocytes that secrete melanin into the hair at the bulb; and second, the hair follicles of Blacks are more helical (spiral) in formation than those of the peoples of other races.

In other words, these helical follicles serve as the spiral corridors from whence the hair leaves the dermis. Hence, before the hair of a Black person even emerges from the scalp, its spiral fashioning has already begun. In that the follicles of other races are not helical—the hair leaves the dermis without spiraling (straighter).

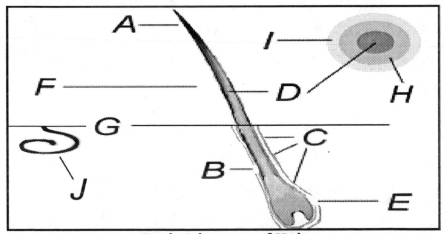

Basic Diagram of Hair
A. Hair B. Root C. Follicle D. Medulla E. Bulb F. Shaft G. Dermis (skin) H. Fibrous Cortex I. Cuticle J. Black Follicle

Why Black Hair Locks

The <u>medulla</u> extends through the center of the hair from the bulb to the end of its shaft and is hollow and contains air. It is encased by a structure known as the <u>fibrous cortex</u>. The fibrous cortex in turn is encased by the <u>cuticle</u> or outermost part of the hair. Melanocytes stored in the follicle secrete activated melanin into the cortex.[3] We've already discussed the fact that activated melanin provides color to the skin—the more the richer—well, it also plays an important role in the locking process of Black hair!

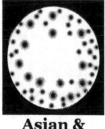

Asian & Nat/Amer

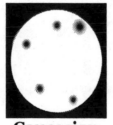

Caucasian

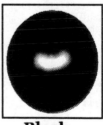

Black

---

[3] Ryder, M., <u>Hair</u> p. 4 & Hair, <u>Collier's Encyclopedia</u> Vol. XI, pp. 579 – 580 & Hair (Human): Structure, Function, Shape, and Growth <u>Human Physiology On File, New Edition 2003</u> Facts On File, Inc. (net) & Hair and its Structure, <u>stophairlossnow</u> 2006 (net) & Hair Analysis, <u>Bergen County Technical Schools</u> (net) & Hair, <u>Animal Diversity Web</u> 2006 (net)

The preceding diagram represents the relative melanin and air content inside the cortex and medulla of the different races of man. In the case of the Yellow and Red Races, this part of the hair contains enough melanin to produce its dark color. In the case of the Caucasian Race, the cortex has relatively little melanin. On the other hand, amongst Blacks we find this part of the hair to be completely saturated with activated melanin. In fact, while the hair shafts of other races appear oval—the melanin content is so great in the hair shaft of the Black Race that the walls of the hair's structures are often stretched to such an extent that they flatten and begin to take on more of a kidney shape.[4]

---

[4] Hair, Encyclopedia Americana Vol. XIII, p. 690 & Hair, Collier's Encyclopedia Vol. XI, pp. 579 - 580 & Hair, The World Book Encyclopedia Vol. IX, p. 9 & Kephart, C., Races of Mankind pp. 55 - 56, 66 & (Video), The Living Body: Skin Deep

Incidentally, the gray or white hair of older people is the result of less melanin in the hair. In addition, the amount of melanin in the hair is thought to enhance the shaft's elasticity; this is probably also true of the skin.

Why Black Hair Locks

To sum this all up, generally speaking, human hair (regardless of race) is made up of five elements: 43% carbon; 31% oxygen; 14.5% nitrogen; 6.5% hydrogen; and 5% sulfur. However, the melanin content within the hair shaft and follicle design varies amongst the races. Thus, it is safe to conclude that it is the helical follicles, coupled with the great amount of activated melanin in every hair shaft, that causes our hair's color (hues most often from black to gold in the young and healthy) resilience, strength, weight, and ability to spiral and lock.[5]

---

[5] Kephart, C., Races of Mankind p. 55, 66 & Coon, C., Racial Adaptations pp. 64 – 65 & Montagu, A., The Concept of Race pp. 122 – 123 & Lillyquist, M., Sunlight & Health: The Positive and Negative Effects of the Sun on You pp. 53 - 54, 67 & New Science: The Last Word – Wave Front (net)
It is possible that the melanin's reaction with the ultraviolet rays of the sun also plays a part in the hair's circular growth pattern. It is noteworthy that different parts of the body are known to absorb the varying properties of sunlight. For example, Lillyquist explains: *"To have an impact on the cell of an organism, sunlight must first be absorbed instead of being reflected or transmitted . . . Different molecules absorb only certain wavelengths of radiation [i.e., the physiological*

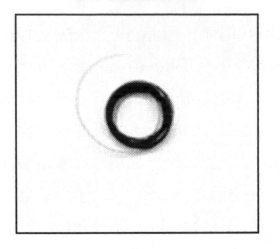

This blown-up image is of a hair at the very tip (or end) of a long lock that's been trimmed. I am showing it to you because even after several years, the hair's tight circular shape is just as clear and fixed now as when it was first grown! Once more then—the hair being formed early on by the follicle, coupled with its heavy melanin

---

benefits from sunlight on the skin are different from sunlight entering the eyes], and as they do they are activated or excited. A chemical change in the molecule may be the result, or the radiation may be reemitted as radiation of longer wavelengths or as heat. Vision is a prime example of a chemical change induced by light. As light strikes our retina, pigment in the receptor cells of the retina absorbs it and communicates the information to the brain by means of electrical and chemical changes . . ."

content (actually causing its structural walls to bulge), work together to make and hold the hair's spiral (or ringlet) shape. Hence, it's the steady procession of this pre-ordained circling in the hair of the Black Race that causes it to naturally gather and ultimately lock!

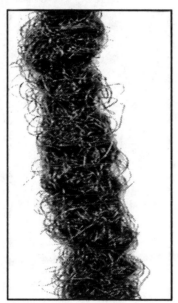

This is a <u>discarded</u> lock that's about 7 inches long (its fraying is due to not being oiled or kept). Yet, what's interesting is that while many of the Blacks who put dangerous chemicals on their hair are unable to grow a single hair shaft 5 or 6 inches long—blacks with locking hair can throw away much more hair than that (7 inches in this case) and not even miss it!

Where
There is no true Self-Comprehension
There can be no genuine Self-Respect

Because the ancient Egyptians appreciated their biology—they were able to grow their hair long and in many naturally locking and attractive styles. Conversely, many Blacks in these times do not have a grasp of their biology and attempt to make their hair long through some kind of traumatic straightening process. However, just as by definition a circle is not straight—the hair shafts are soon damaged to such an extent that they must break off. Thus, what many might consider long Black hair today would be short in the eyes of the ancients.

Look, I am a student of history who has done research around the world. Believe me, there are a myriad of subjects I'd rather be discussing with you; however, the principal reason for my penning this work is summed up by these words about a recent study of hair loss in African American women:

"For many sisters the price of looking cute [having hair that's straight] has become too high a price to pay. For there is increasing evidence that too tight braids, ponytails or extensions, bonding glue, chemical relaxers and layering of multiple hair treatments are among the most common reasons for hair loss in African American women. The problem affects an estimated 22 million women in the United States, often creating self-esteem issues and causing severe depression . . ."[1]

Have you caught the irony—in attempting to "correct" their God-given biology and make their ulotrichous (spiral and locking) hair straight and long—in the short term they cause it to break off and in the long—they create such damage to their hair and scalp that they contribute to their

---

[1] Health Hotline: Hairloss Ebony Vol. LIX, No. 12 Oct. 2004 p. 85 (net)

<u>own balding</u>! This is far removed understanding of their foremothers w... that a woman's natural hair was an aspect of her glory. Yet, we needn't be surprised by this African American dilemma considering the nation's history. That said, <u>until you respect your nature—your nature cannot respect you</u>!

The fact of the matter is as long as a Black person's heart beats—activated melanin will be secreted into, and spirally shape, his or her hair. All of the tales about salt water, wax molds, twisting, and not washing Black hair to make it lock—<u>are false</u>. In fact, some of these notions are rather silly considering that the no people placed more importance on hygiene than the ancient Egyptians! In truth, the adage: *"Cleanliness is next to Godliness"* came from ancient Egypt! What's more, Egypt's lock wearing women were distinguished for their hygienic habits—from the washing, styling and

.he oiling of their hair; to the painting of their finger and toe nails; to the use of kohl (eye liner), deodorants and perfumes. Frankly, the Black women of ancient Egypt were the standard of beauty for the peoples of the Old World! [2]

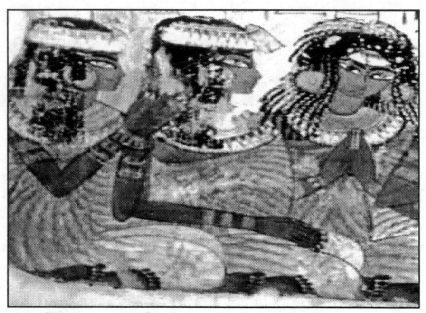

Egyptian women during a festive occasion c.1400 BC

[2] Burn, A., & Selincourt, A., Herodotus: The Histories p. 143 & (Video), Ancient Lives WTTW 1988 & David, R., The Egyptian Kingdoms pp. 115 - 116 & Velikovsky, I., Ramses II and his Time & Budge, E.A., The Dwellers on the Nile p. 71, 74 & Mialon, E., The Great Pharaoh Ramses and His Time Chp. 61 & Ghalioungui, P., Magic and Medical Science in ancient Egypt p. 152 & Hobson, C., The World of the Pharaohs & Duckat, W., Beggar to King pp. 5 - 8 & Health Hotline: Hairloss Ebony Vol. LIX, No. 12 Oct. 2004 p. 85

A Circle in Time

It is clear that the ancients did not have an aversion to the idea of a circle being anatomically expressed through their hair. You see, in the Old World the circle was a profound symbol: for example, (1) the Egyptian God Thoth spoke of the circular operations of the neters; (2) the Mansion of Eternity was thought to be round; (3) some spiritual dances were performed in the round; (4) the Egyptians understood that the earth was round and that planets moved in a circular motion; (5) indeed Time itself was said to function as a circle; and (6), the circle was representative of beginning without end.

Additionally, we find this reverence for the circle present in other parts of the Old World. For instance, the circle was a centerpiece of ancient Babylonian art. The Chakra of Buddhists (symbolic of the universal life system) is depicted as a circle or wheel. We even find modern scientists theorizing that the course of the universe is cyclical. To quote Goodman: *"Without doubt, the circle is the most important of all units in magical symbolism, and in almost every case where it is used, the circle is intended to denote spirit, or spiritual forces."*

But atop all this, biologists studying the human genome explain that the spherical pattern is found when examining the essence of human life. That's right; DNA molecules are structured so as to form a double helix (or two spirals).

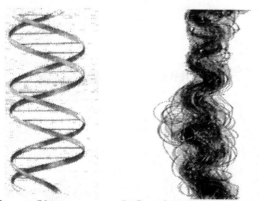

The left is a diagram of the human DNA Helix. The right is 2" of the end of a <u>discarded</u> lock (the obvious fraying is from not being oiled). Yet, the similarity between the DNA Helix and the natural helical pattern of the lock is instantly recognizable.

DNA aside here, coming to such understanding about the ancients makes it rather easy to see why a spiritual people would embrace their locking spirals (see "J" page 34). They are another wonderful expression of man's relationship to the creation. What's more, why should anyone who claims to love the Creator object to this omnipresent pattern being incorporated into an important aspect of their physical being? Indeed, forasmuch as the body has been declared a temple—those who disown this aspect of their nature are rejecting the work of their Divine Maker![1]

---

[1] Goodman, F., Magic Symbols pp. 16 – 17 & Ward, P., A Dictionary of Common Fallacies p. 2 & Quirke, S., Ancient Egyptian Religion p. 26 & Hermes Mercurius Trismegistus: his Divine Pymander in Seventeen Books Bk. III & Hall, M., The Secret Teachings of All Ages p. XCIII & Tompkins, P., The Magic of Obelisks pp. 350 - 353 & Meyer, M., The Gnostic Gospels of Jesus & Oates, J., Babylon p. 198 & Schulberg, L., Historic India & (Video), Transformation of Myth Through Time: From Psychology to Spirituality W. Free 1989 & Bunson, M., A Dictionary of Ancient Egypt p. 86 & Image credit: U.S. Department of Energy Human Genome Program (net) & John 2:19-22
The Christ's words were: *"Destroy this temple, and in three days I will raise it up."*

Racism & Hair

Let me be as clear as I can—<u>any Black infatuation with possessing straight hair on this planet is a very late phenomenon</u>! The root of this self-rejection is White (Western) racism and all of the aspersions made by (for lack of a better phrase) the "Humanely Challenged" about the anatomy of the Black Race. Unfortunately, it is an artifice that has scared the psyche of millions of African Americans.

By contrast—and against the back drop of the racism and dehumanizing insults African Americans encounter today—one cannot help note that by the time Egyptian children were school age they were aware that straight hair and bodies that were not actively melanized (pale to pinkish) are biological traits found amongst the lower primates. In fact, Charles Darwin was to explain that this point of view has been held in Africa through the millennia.

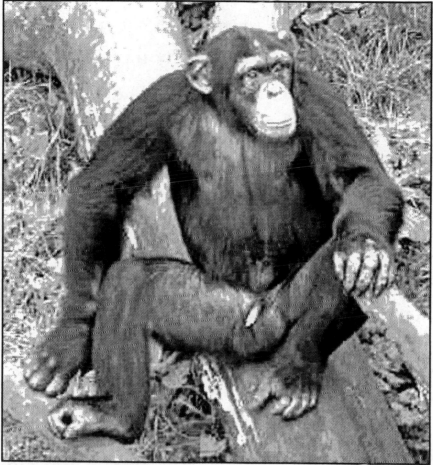

Primates are divided into two basic classifications. The lower classification is called Prosimians and consists of the lemur, loris and some tree shrews. The higher classification is called Anthropoids and is comprised of monkeys, apes, and humans. Of the apes, it is the chimpanzee (pictured) that comes closest to human beings genetically. Incredibly, chimps share more genetic material with humans than they do with gorillas.

Photo appears courtesy ZOO Liberec

In truth, Western anthropologists have been making the point since the early 1900s that even though great apes are found in geographical regions that African peoples inhabit—the hair of these primates (great apes) is not helical or locking like the hair of the African Race. For instance, in a discussion of the hair of humans and great apes, on page 824 of the XII Volume of the 11th Edition of the Encyclopaedia Britannica we find: *"Thus, the white races are seen to come nearest the higher apes in this respect, yellow next, and black farthest removed."*

This shared; my point here is not that Whites have more biological traits in common with apes than Blacks or vice-versa. The species of Homo-Sapien Sapien is Homo-Sapien Sapien; nothing more, nothing less—the scriptures even attests to this fact! Truthfully, the point here is this:

Racism & Hair

"Where personal self respect wanes, so must happiness."[1]

As previously stated, the application of harsh chemicals to straighten and/or color Black hair commonly retards its growth and causes breakage. Some of these treatments even cause such detrimental results as premature balding, nerve damage and possibly even birth defects. I realize that old habits can be hard to break; but to sadomasochistically embrace this Euro-Indoctrination can only lead to the domain of the <u>Indoctro-Niggated</u>: i.e., Black beauty,

---

[1] Milele, N., <u>The Journey of the Songhai People</u> p. 31 & Hartman, H., <u>The great Ages</u> The Factmonster (net) 2006 & (Video), <u>The Living Body: Skin Deep</u> & Montagu, A., <u>Man's Most Dangerous Myth: The Fallacy of Race</u> p. 95 & (Video), <u>The Science of Sex: The Aim of the Game</u> 1998 & <u>Genesis</u> 1:24-27 & <u>I Corinthians</u> 15:39 & <u>Acts</u> 17:26 & Human Beings, <u>Encyclopedia Americana</u> Vol. XIV, pp. 545 - 546 & <u>Cambridge Encyclopedia of Human Evolution</u> p. 274 & Races of Man, <u>The World Book Encyclopedia</u> Vol. XIV, p. 6732 & Rogers, J.A., <u>Sex and Race</u> Vol. I, p. 78, Vol. II, pp. 402 – 403

I believe that the aforementioned quote should either be attributed to Henry David Thoreau or Walt Whitman.

creativity, intellect and achievement always being depicted as substandard to people of other races.

The belief that there is something innately undesirable with your Black physiology (i.e., hair and skin) is nothing but an underpinning for the pathology of self-hate. Look, racist supermarket or not—*there's no law that says you have to buy what they're sellin!* As for what to do if you're someone who's struggling, a good start would be to embrace these words by Matthew Maltz:

> *See yourself in a new light, as an*
> *individual like no one else on earth . . .*
> *Believe in this new truth, and act on it!*
> *Resolve to be your own friend, not your*
> *enemy!*"[2]

---

[2] Maltz, M., The Magic Power of Self-Image Psychology pp. 4 - 11, 18 - 19 & Rogers, J.A., World's Great Men of Color Vol. I, pp. 92 - 93
Even while your humanity is being maligned in every quarter in these times—you must reject self-hate at all cost! The reason is simple, hate only leads to death . . .

Racism & Hair

Simply stated, our ancestors abided a genuine reality. Consequently, they would not be vulnerable to the devices of anyone whose only aim was to divorce them from themselves. What's more, holding the Creator and his gifts in reverence—it would be unthinkable for an ancient "Child of the Light" to reject their highly melanized skin and hair. Thus, employing negative connotations to describe their naturally locking hair would not occupy even a miniscule part of the ancient African psyche!

Once again, I must applaud our ancestors for not only dwelling in the realm of self-love—but for understanding that to not possess activated melanin is nothing more, or less, than it is. Yet and still, the ancient Egyptian word for their hair was *"Sent"* and its hieroglyphic symbol was a black shaft with a curl at the end.[iii]

Hieroglyph

Real Lock

Growth, Care & Maintenance

I won't spend a lot of time discussing the "Afro" or "Natural" hairstyle. As it was the predominate hairstyle of African Americans a generation ago, most of you either wore, or have a friend and/or family member who could help you to get your "fro" together.

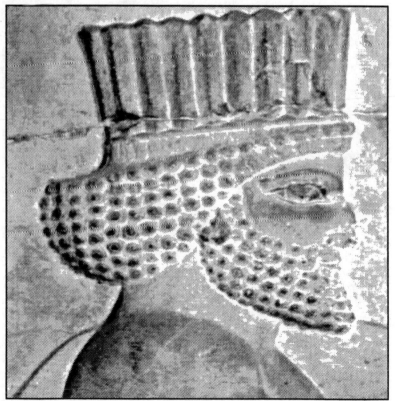

Black Mesopotamian Soldier. This stone artifact is almost 3000 years old (also see back cover)

We have already seen that the ringlet or circular character has been predetermined for the Black hair shaft before it emerges from the skin (pages 34 – 37). This means that any kind of twisting, braiding, or epic measure like importing ocean water from Jamaica is pointless. Indeed, 90% of the time the more incredible and expensive the exercise—the less effective it proves. The surest way for most Black people to make sure that their hair will lock is to not perform any ambitious manipulation to it whatsoever.

As for how long it will take to grow a full head of locks—everyone's hair grows at different rates according to the individual's physiology, diet and overall health. However, if a Black person was to ask me what to do to grow locks, this is what I would tell them:

- Cut your chemically treated hair off; not only is there a strong likelihood that its severely damaged—but its natural rings, which are the essence of each lock, have already been compromised. So I would recommend cutting the hair as close as you're comfortable with. If you don't have treated hair that's better for producing new locks; however, if you've been pickin, raking or combing it, I'd still suggest cutting it as close as your comfortable with. The idea here is that virgin shafts look the best and have the best chance of reaching maturity.

- So, starting with a clean slate (hair cut as close as you're comfortable with) here's where the fun starts. Your mission—should you choose to accept it—is to shampoo with any off of the shelf inexpensive drugstore shampoo and conditioner as often as you can. The greater the frequency the better in the beginning because the water and shampooing are stimulating to the scalp and hair.

- The other important part of the process is to liberally apply (warm to the touch not cold) olive oil to your hair. The amount of oil will vary depending upon the length and thickness of your locking hair. Once more, the oil is stimulating to the hair and will also soften and make your locks more pliable. Oiling your locks will also reduce fraying. You want to apply oil to each lock but not so much that its drippy. I would do this once a week or so at the start. FYI: olive oil can be tough to wash out of some clothing items so approach its application the way you would washing your hair. For example, on a lazy day you could thoroughly massage and oil your scalp and locks in the morning. Throw on an old sweat-shirt and go on about your day. That evening, use the same inexpensive shampoo and conditioner you've been using all week to wash the oil out—and you're through! After your locks have come in and are established, you can decide when to apply the warm olive oil treatments according to the texture. Here, I'm reminded of the passage: *You anoint my head with oil, my cup runneth over . . ."*

- Your individual ringlets will grow and before long begin to gather and become locks. Now this is the period when the overall picture of your hair can be unruly. Word: your head is your head and your locks are your locks—but if you wish, you can bring some uniformity to your locks by simply taking the thumbs and fore fingers of both hands and pulling small areas of locks apart from one another. Short virgin locks stand up straight from the scalp. However, as your locks get longer and heavier they will lie down (e.g., like in many of the portraits in this book).

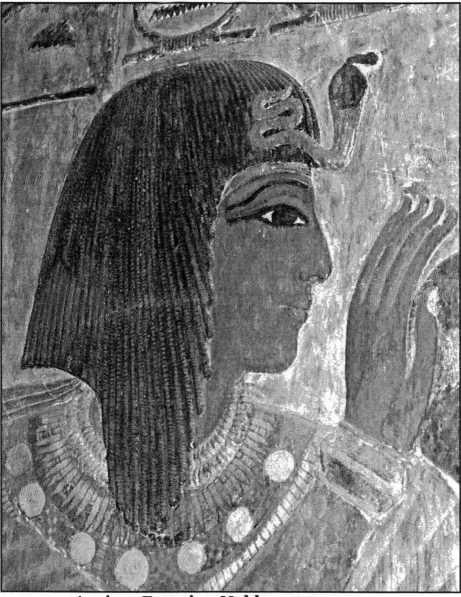

Ancient Egyptian Nobleman c.1100

- Black locks can be cut with a pair of scissors to
  any length or style you wish. If you'd like,
  start with one of the styles in this book—and

ladies, I'm sure you won't have any problem coming up with many of your own!

- If you're an independent person who's on the fence about permitting your hair to lock, let me leave you with the worst that can happen should you try it: you'll save money; you won't be putting harsh, smelly or poisonous chemicals on, or into, your body; you won't be doing anything that will lead to premature baldness or scalp damage; you won't be at risk for burning; you'll be creating more time in your life for other things; and, you're going to look a whole lot better in my estimation!

- Lastly, if you'd like to wear your hair in the healthy and natural way that its been worn by your people for millenniums but you're worried about employer harassment—that could be a real concern. But should you decide not to let any employer control how you walk through life or come between you and yourself—<u>sue any employer</u> who harasses you for making the personal decision to stop assaulting your own anatomy and health![1] Just make sure that your attorney gets a copy of this book before the trial.

---

[1] How appropriate that a dangerous chemical known as <u>lye</u> should be used to straighten the hair of African Americans.

Lost & Found

Look, as student of history who has studied our experience on this planet for decades—I am convinced that the keys to our future do not lie with others, but rest within ourselves! If the truth is to be told, no race has had a greater history or given more to the world than our branch of humanity.

Additionally, when it comes to our physiology, here too, we have nothing to be ashamed of, or to feel insecure about—from the anatomical structure of our bodies from our limbs to our brains—the Creator has not cheated us in any way! Anyone with a modicum of knowledge about the history of this planet would know this.

However, just in case you've been left out of the loop and haven't received the word, allow me to take a moment to help bring you up to speed. Just briefly here, in his assessment of the contribution of the Black Race to Old World civilization, Daniel would remark:

"European history begins with a paradox: what we regard as indispensable preconditions for Western civilization first appear not within the geographic confines of Europe but in the Near East, in Mesopotamia and Egypt, between 4000 and 3000 B.C. . . . We can view these Near Eastern societies of the post-neolithic era as the starting point for European history even though it was not until after 1450 BC. that a society anywhere approximating this level of civilization appeared within the geographical limits of Europe . . ."[1]

---

[1] <u>Ancient Civilization: 4000 B.C. - 400 A.D.</u> p. 4
Daniel is underscoring the fact that attempting to portray the Greek culture as developing independent of earlier Black civilization is not possible.

So, in closing, let me leave you with this to smoke over. Were an ancient Black person of the Fertile Crescent able to come to this time and canvass the African American community, he (or she) would no doubt have many questions. However, one question they would not have to ask is why have a small number of African Americans chosen to wear their hair in locks. Rather, it is much more likely that they would want to know why most do not?[2]

If you will know yourselves, then you will be known and you will know that you are the children of the Living Father. But if you do not know yourselves, then you are in poverty and you are poverty . . .

Yeshua Ham-Mashiach

---

[2] Luke 19:10

For generations now, Blacks have understood that there's a big difference between an African American and one of America's Africans. I hope that this is not wasted on you because while it's true that the Son of Man came to seek out and save that which is lost—there is a vast difference between that which is lost and that which chooses to be missing!

Lost & Found

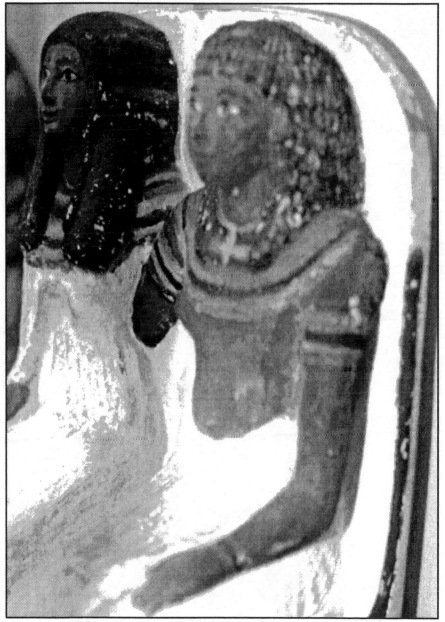

Noble Couple of Ancient Egypt c. 1400 BC

Epilogue

Epilogue

*W*hile some of you know my voice, many of you do not. This effort has not been made so that you would call yourselves Egyptians. The book was not authored so that you would call yourselves Jews or Ishmailites. It was not made to create friction between those with understanding and those without. Lastly, it was not written so that you would be more like me. The reason that this effort was made was so that You might ultimately be more like You . . .

Peace -

R.L.

Endnotes

Endnotes for "Locks"

i. Gaskell, G., <u>Dictionary of all Scriptures and Myths</u> & Murphy, E., <u>Diodorus on Egypt</u> p. 22 & Bunson, M., <u>A Dictionary of Ancient Egypt</u> p. 29 & Muller, M., <u>Mythology of All Races</u> Vol. XII, p. 202 & Dodson, A., <u>Monarchs of the Nile</u> p. 102 & Reeves, N., <u>Into the Mummy's Tomb</u> p. 61 & Budge, E.A., <u>A History of Egypt</u> Vol. I, p. 29, 86 & Trigger, B., Kemp, B., O' Connor, D., & Lloyd, A., <u>Ancient Egypt: A Social History</u> p. 59 & Mertz, B., <u>Red Land, Black Land</u> p. 79 & Gordon, C., <u>Before the Bible</u> p. 62 & Whiston, W., <u>The Life and Works of Flavius Josephus</u> p. 119 & <u>Numbers</u> 6:5 & <u>Judges</u> 13:5, Chp. 16 & <u>The Song of Songs</u> 5:2-12 & Epstein, L., <u>Sex, Laws, and Customs in Judaism</u> & McCray, W., <u>The Black Presence in the Bible: Discovering the Black and African Identity of Biblical Persons and Nations</u> & <u>Illustrated Dictionary & Concordance of the Bible</u> p. 874 & <u>I Corinthians</u> 11:2-15 & <u>Daniel</u> 7:9 & <u>Revelations</u> 1:14 & Walker, B., <u>The Woman's Encyclopedia of Myths and Secrets</u> & Owen, F., <u>The Germanic People</u> p. 117 & Hairdressing, <u>The American Peoples Encyclopedia</u> Vol. X & <u>Numbers</u> 6:5-10 & Burn, A., & Selincourt, A., <u>Herodotus: The Histories</u> pp. 281 - 282 & Grimal, P., <u>Dictionary of Classical Mythology</u> p. 311 & <u>Ezekiel</u> 8:3 & Waszink, J., <u>De Anima</u> p. 445

*The ancient Hebrews also cut their hair in times of mourning.

*Amongst some ancient societies beards were symbolic of the attainment of spiritual wisdom.

*I know that many of you believe that the ancient Hebrews were Caucasian—that's false. In brief, Judaism is a religion that's been practiced by people of all races in the later ages. However, the Hebrew Patriarch Abraham and his immediate descendents were born, and spent their entire lives, in the Fertile Crescent—which in his day was inhabited and dominated by Blacks.

*Egypt's rulers often wore a false beard during ceremony.

*In passing, a person's locks could also be cut and sacrificed in burnt offerings to the gods. In such cases it was the smoke of the sacrifice that was prayed to be received.

*In many instances amongst the Hebrews, locks were a type of crown for men that were not to be cut before

Endnotes

the holy consecration—and a woman's locks were an aspect of her glory!

*Even amongst the Celts of Europe, short hair was only worn by the young or criminals.

Endnotes for "Why Black Hair Locks"

i. Biological Coloration, The Encyclopedia Britannica Vol. XVI, p. 588 & Sek-kem, G., Melanin and the Next Millennium: The Kem-Wer Factor & Coon, C., Racial Adaptations pp. 48 – 51 & Wills, C., The Skin We're In Discover Nov. 15, No. 11 Nov. 1994 pp. 79, 80 - 81 & Milele, N., The Journey of the Songhai People pp. 46 – 51 & Pierpaoli, W., Regelson, W., & Colman, C., The Melatonin Miracle pp. 70 - 73 & (Video), The Living Body: Skin Deep & Hall, M., The Secret Teachings of All Ages p. LXXIX & Coon, C., Contemporary Authors Vol. 104, p. 91 & Rogers, J.A., Sex and Race Vol. I, p. 276, Vol. III, p. 136 & Budge, E.A., A History of Ethiopia p. 5 & Higgins, G., Anacalypsis Vol. II, p. 136 & Quirke, S., & Spencer, J., The British Museum Book of Ancient Egypt p. 220 & Muller, M., Mythology of All Races Vol. XII, pp. 96 – 97, Vol. XII, p. 386 & Jobes, G., Dictionary of Mythology, Folklore and Symbols p. 1314 & Tompkins, P., The Magic of Obelisks p. 441 &

Budge, E.A., <u>The Book of the Dead</u> p. 505 & Gaskell, G., <u>Dictionary of all Scriptures and Myths</u> p. 38, 319, 554 & Foster, J., <u>Love Songs of the New Kingdom</u> & Hall, M. <u>The Secret Teachings of All Ages</u> p. XLVI & Reeves, N., <u>Into the Mummy's Tomb</u> p. 47 & Van Sertima, I., <u>Blacks in Science: ancient and modern</u> p. 34 & <u>The Lost Books of the Bible and the Forgotten Books of Eden</u> p. 211 & <u>Revelation</u> 3:18 & <u>II Timothy 2:20</u>

*Researchers explain:

> *"There are two types of melanin: eumelanin (black melanin), and phaeomelanin (dun, or orange to red melanin) . . . A granule of either type of melanin starts out as a colorless ball inside a membranous container. If destined to become eumelanin, it turns into a flattish oval body with concentric laminations. As time goes on, it begins to become pigmented and its structure becomes blurred, unless it is a dud— scheduled to remain colorless. Fully ripened granules are flat, blackish discs between 1.3 and 1.0 microns long and between 0.6 and 0.5 microns wide."*

Endnotes

*Albinos possess the least amount of activated melanin. Unfortunately, they are faced with a myriad of illnesses that other populations are not.

*Parenthetically, scientists explain that the Black Race has a lower incidence of Parkinson's Disease than the other races.

*It is also possible that the brain's ability to produce dopamine is a factor in performing complex movement fluently.

*That aside, the ancient Egyptians associated the pineal gland with Ra.

*The Egyptians saw gold as the state where wisdom and truth were clearly perceived. Osiris' color was originally black. Once obtaining his higher state he turned gold. In passing, gold is also thought to have been used in the restoration of the deity's body after his death.

*An expression of this concept is also expressed biblically in The Song of Solomon. In Chapter 1:5-6 we find: *"I am black, but comely. . . Look not upon me, because I am black . . ."* Then in chapter 5:11 it is explained: *"His head is as the most fine gold . . ."*

And in Timothy we read: *"But in a great house there are not only vessels of gold and silver, but also of wood and earth . . ."*

Endnotes for "Racism & Hair"

iii. Budge, E.A., <u>Egyptian Language</u> p. 55 & Nichols, T., <u>Rastafari</u> & Budge, E.A., <u>The Book of the Dead</u> p. 205, 260 Budge, E.A., <u>A History of Ethiopia</u> p. 123 & Higgins, G., <u>Anacalypsis</u> Vol. I, p. 769 & <u>I Samuel</u> 16:4 & Whiston, W., <u>The Life and Works of Flavius Josephus</u> p. 119, 164 & <u>Judges</u> 16:17-19 & Rogers, J.A., <u>Sex and Race</u> Vol. I, p. 30

*As mentioned, Blacks have worn locks throughout antiquity. However, with the Rastafarian movement in Jamaica during the 20th century, people of this era commonly refer to the locking hair of Blacks as "Dread Locks." The term "Rastafarian" stems from the man Ras Tafari who's known to the world as the Ethiopian Emperor Halie Selassie I. Rastafarians believe locks to be an essential feature of their

Endnotes

spiritual growth. Rastas further explain that the term "Dreads" originated in ancient times amongst those who feared the power that was associated with the lock wearing Prophets of Yahweh! As it was written in the account of Samson and Delilah:

"He told her all his heart, and said to her, There hath not come a razor upon mine head; for I have been a Nazarite unto God from my mother's womb: if I be shaven then my strength will go from me . . . And she made him sleep upon her knees; and she called for a man, and she caused him to shave off the seven locks of his head . . ."

Bibliography

Bibliography

Boorstin, D., The Discoverers Random House 1985

Budge, E.A., A History of Egypt Anthropological Pub. 1968

Budge, E.A., A History of Ethiopia Anthropological Pub. 1966

Budge, E.A., Egypt Holt 1925

Budge, E.A., Egyptian Language Routledge & Paul 1963

Budge, E.A., The Book of the Dead Univ. Books 1960

Budge, E.A., The Book of the Dead Arkana 1985

Budge, E.A., The Book of the Dead Carol Publ. 1994

Budge, E.A., The Dwellers on the Nile Dover 1977

Bullock, M., Daily Life in Ancient Egypt McGraw Hill 1964

Bunson, M., A Dictionary of Ancient Egypt Oxford Univ. 1995

Burn, A., & Selincourt, A., Herodotus the Histories Penguin 1972

Butzer, C. (Ed.)., Ancient Egypt: Discovering Its Splendors National Geographic Soc. 1978

Coon, C., Racial Adaptations Nelson – Hall 1982

David, R., The Egyptian Kingdoms Elsevier & Phaidon 1975

Dodson, A., Monarchs of the Nile Rubicon Press 1995

Duckat, W., Beggar to King Doubleday 1968

Eban, A., Heritage: Civilization and the Jews Summit Books 1984

Epstein, L., Sex Laws and Customs in Judaism Bloch Publ. 1948

Freemantle, A., A Treasury of Early Christianity Viking 1953

Gaskell, G., Dictionary of all Scriptures and Myths Julien Press 1960

Ghalioungui, P., Magic and Medical Science in Ancient Egypt Barnes & Noble 1963

Glubot, S., Discovering the Royal Tombs at Ur Macmillan 1969

Goodman, F., Magic Symbols Trodd Publ. House 1989

Gordon, C., Before the Bible Harper & Row 1962

Gray, J., Near Eastern Mythology Bedrick 1985

Grimal, P., The Dictionary of Classical Mythology Blackwell 1985

Hall, M., The Secret Teachings of All Ages The Philosophical Research Soc. 1977

Bibliography

Hartman, H., The great Ages The Factmonster
http://www.factmonster.com/spot/ape1.html 2006
Herm, G., Phoenicians Morrow 1975
Higgins, G., Anacalypsis University Books 1965
Hobson, C., The World of the Pharaohs Thames &
Hudson 1982
Jobes, G., Dictionary of Mythology, Folklore and
Symbols Scarecrow Publ. 1961
Kephart, C., Races of Mankind N.Y. Philosophical
Lib. 1960
Lillyquist, M., Sunlight & Health: The Positive and
Negative Effects of the Sun on You Dodd, Mead &
Co. 1985
Lucas, A., Ancient Egyptian Materials & Industry
E. Arnold Co. 1926
Macaulay, R., Pleasure of Ruins Thames and
Hudson 1964
Maltz, M., The Magic Power of Self-Image
Psychology Pocket Books 1970
McCray, W., The Black Presence in the Bible Black
Light Fellowship 1990
Mertz, B., Red Land, Black Land McCann 1966
Meyer, M., The Gnostic Gospels of Jesus
HarperCollins 2005

Mialon, E., The Great Pharaoh Ramses and His Time Exim Publ. 1985

Milele, N., The Journey of the Songhai People Pan African Fed. 1987

Montagu, A., Man's Most Dangerous Myth: The Fallacy of Race The World Publ. Co. 1964

Montagu, A., The Concept of Race Free Press 1964

Muller, M., Mythology of All Races Vol. XII Cooper Square 1964

Murphy, E., Diodorus on Egypt McFarland 1985

Nichols, T., Rastifari Doubleday 1979

Oates, J., Babylon Thames & Hudson 1979

Owen, F., The Germanic People Bookman Assoc. 1960

Pierpaoli, W., Regelson, W., & Colman, C., The Melatonin Miracle: Nature's Age-Reversing, Disease-Fighting, Sex-Enhancing Hormone Simon & Schuster 1995

Quirke, S., Ancient Egyptian Religion Dover 1992

Quirke, S., & Spencer, J., The British Museum Book of Ancient Egypt Thames & Hudson 1992

Reeves, N., Into the Mummy's Tomb Madison Press 1992

Robinson, C., Conversion of Europe Longman, Green & Co. 1917

Bibliography

Rogers, J.A., Sex and Race Rogers Publ. 1967

Rogers, J.A., World's Great Men of Color Macmillan 1972

Ryder, M., Hair Arnold Publ. 1973

Schulberg, L., Historic India Time 1968

Scullard, H., Roman Britain Thames & Hudson 1979

Sek-kem, G., Melanin and the Next Millennium: The Kem-Wer Factor (Notes of 2nd Annual Kem-Wer Conference 1987) Sek-Kem 1988

Simons, G., Barbarian Europe Timelife 1968

Tompkins, P., The Magic of Obelisks Harper & Row 1981

Van Sertima, I., Blacks in Science: Ancient and Modern Transactions 1983

Velikovsky, I., Rameses II and his Time Doubleday 1978

Ward, P., A Dictionary of Common Fallacies Prometheus Books 1989

Wheeler, M., Flames Over Persepolis Reynal Co. 1968

Wheelwright, E., Medicinal Plants and their History Dover 1974

_____., Ancient Civilization: 4000 B.C. - 400 A.D. T.Y. Crowell 1972

_____., Ancient Egypt: A Social History Cambridge Univ. 1983

_____., Ancient Lives (Video) Spry-Leverton & WTTW 1984, 1988

_____., Ancient Mesopotamia Nauka Publ. 1969

_____., Cambridge Encyclopedia of Human Evolution Cambridge Univ. Press 1992

_____., Collier's Encyclopedia Macmillan 1986

_____., Contemporary Authors Gale Research 1982

_____., Encyclopaedia Britannica Encyclopaedia Britannica Inc. 1999 - 2002

_____., Encyclopedia Americana Grolier Publ. 2001

_____., Great Soviet Encyclopedia Macmillan 1985

Hair Analysis, Bergen County Technical Schools 2006 http://www.bergen.org/EST/Year5/HairAnalysis.htm

Hair and its Structure, Stophairlossnow (2006) http://www.stophairlossnow.com/Hair%20Structure.htm

Bibliography

Hair, Animal Diversity Web Univ. of Mich. Museum of Zoology (2006) http://animaldiversity.ummz.umich.edu/ site/topics/mammal_anatomy/hair.html

Hair (Human): Structure, Function, Shape, and Growth, Human Physiology On File, New Edition 2003 Facts On File, Inc. (2006) Science Online: www.factsonfile.com

Health Hotline: Hairloss, Ebony Vol. LIX, No. 12 Oct. 2004 p. 85 (2006) http://www.proquest.com

_____., Hermes Mercurius Trismegistus: his Divine Pymander in Seventeen Books T. Brewster 1657

_____., Illustrated Dictionary & Concordance of the Bible Jerusalem Publ. House 1986

Image credit: U.S. Department of Energy Human Genome Program, http://www.ornl.gov/hgmis

_____., New Science: The Last Word – Wave Front http://www.newscientist.com/lastword/ 07-25-02

_____., The American Peoples Encyclopedia Spencer Press 1955

_____., The Living Body: Skin Deep (Video) Films for the Humanities 1985

_____., The Lost Books of the Bible and the Forgotten Books of Eden Bell 1979

_____., The Science of Sex: The Aim of the Game (Video) The Learning Chan. 1998

_____., The World Book Encyclopedia World Book Inc. 1970 – 2003 editions

_____., Transformation of a Myth through Time: Campbell Lecture Series (Video) W. Free 1989

Trigger, B., Kemp, B., O' Connor, D., & Lloyd, A., Walker, B., The Woman's Encyclopedia of Myths and Secrets Rodeo Press 1981

Waszink, J., De Anima Meulenhoff 1947

Whiston, W., The Life and Works of Flavius Josephus Holt, Rinehart & Winston 1957

Wills, C., The Skin We're In Discover Nov. 15, No. 11 Nov. 1994 pp. 80 - 89

Your Notes

About **Black Hair**

Your Notes

About **Black Hair**

Your Notes

About **Black Hair**

Your Notes

<u>About</u> **Black Hair**

Your Notes

About **Black Hair**